CELIAC DISEASE DIET COOKBOOK

Gluten-Free Recipes For Health, Easy Meal Plans, Nutrient-Rich Foods, And Delicious Gluten-Free Dishes

DR ELIAN GRIFFIN

Copyright © [Elian Griffin] [2024]. All rights reserved.

Without the publisher's prior written consent, no portion of this publication may be copied, distributed, or transmitted in any way, including by photocopying, recording, or other mechanical or electronic means, with the exception of brief quotations used in all critical reviews.

DISCLAIMER

The nutritional recommendations and recipes in this book are meant solely for informative reasons. They are not meant to replace the counsel, diagnosis, or care of a qualified medical expert. If you have any doubts about a medical condition or dietary requirements, you should always see your physician or another trained healthcare expert.

All reasonable efforts have been taken by the author and publisher to ensure that the information contained in this book is correct as of the date of publication. Recommendations may alter, though, as medical knowledge is always changing. When using any of the recipes or instructions found here, the user assumes all liability and assumes no risk, whether personal or otherwise. People who have certain dietary requirements or medical issues should speak with a healthcare provider for personalized guidance. The given recipes are only ideas; you may need to adjust them to suit your own nutritional needs, tastes, and tolerances.

When you use this book, you agree to release the publisher, the author, and their representatives from any liability for any claims, damages, liabilities, costs, or expenditures resulting from your use of the book.

TABLE OF CONTENTS

ABOUT THE BOOK

Understanding the celiac disease is the first step toward effective management, and this cookbook begins by defining and providing an overview of the condition, detailing its symptoms and diagnosis, and explaining the significant impact it has on overall health. Emphasizing the importance of diet management and the role of gluten in celiac disease, this section lays a solid foundation for readers to grasp the necessity of dietary adjustments.

The Celiac Disease Diet Cookbook is an essential guide for anyone managing celiac disease, offering comprehensive insights and practical solutions for maintaining a gluten-free lifestyle.

For people with celiac disease, a gluten-free diet is essential, and this cookbook outlines the many advantages of it. It also explains common gluten sources and cross-contamination scenarios, giving readers the information they need to accurately read food labels and carefully consider their nutritional needs.

It also introduces key components of a gluten-free diet, including dairy and dairy substitutes, as well as gluten-free grains, safe starches, and thickeners. Finally, it discusses the significance of including fruits, vegetables, legumes, and flavorful herbs and spices in a gluten-free diet.

A gluten-free kitchen is essential for preventing cross-contamination and guaranteeing safe meal preparation. The book provides helpful tips for meal planning and preparation, easing the transition to a gluten-free lifestyle, and organizing the kitchen, choosing gadgets and tools, and storing gluten-free ingredients. It also addresses cravings, dining out, navigating social situations, and getting emotional and psychological support. Resources and support groups for those who are new to the gluten-free lifestyle are also highlighted.

In addition to a section devoted to snacks and appetizers, the cookbook is filled with recipes. For breakfast, readers can enjoy gluten-free options like bread and pastries, smoothies and juices, cereals, granolas, and egg-based dishes. For lunch, readers can explore sandwiches, wraps, salads, soups, stews, and light, healthy options. For dinner, there are main courses, side dishes, one-pot meals, casseroles, and family-friendly recipes.

This cookbook offers a variety of recipes for bread, rolls, cakes, cookies, brownies, pies, and pastries, as well as tips for successful gluten-free baking. Since maintaining a gluten-free lifestyle is a journey, it also covers long-term dietary strategies, coping with challenges, staying informed about gluten-free trends, and accessing ongoing support and resources.

Baking without gluten is made easy with this cookbook's guidance on using gluten-free flour and substitutes.

This thorough approach makes the "Celiac Disease Diet Cookbook" an invaluable resource for anyone committed to a healthier, gluten-free life. To ensure readers have all the information they need, the cookbook includes a detailed FAQ section that addresses common concerns like identifying symptoms, ensuring food is truly gluten-free, handling accidental gluten consumption, recognizing gluten-free certifications, and supporting family members with celiac disease.

CHAPTER ONE

DEFINITION AND SYNOPSIS

Gluten, a protein present in wheat, barley, and rye, causes an immune reaction that damages the lining of the small intestine, impairing nutritional absorption and resulting in a host of health problems. The only known treatment for celiac disease is a strict, lifelong gluten-free diet that eliminates all gluten-containing foods and ingredients, allowing those who have the condition to manage their symptoms and lead healthy lives.

The disease can start at any age, and there is a wide range of symptoms that can occur. For example, some people may have very severe digestive problems, while others may not have any gastrointestinal symptoms at all. The disease can also cause non-digestive symptoms like anemia, osteoporosis, and neurological disorders. Due to this wide range of symptoms, celiac disease is frequently misdiagnosed or underdiagnosed, so patients and healthcare professionals need to be aware of the condition.

A thorough understanding of celiac disease and a dedication to following a gluten-free diet are necessary for living with the condition. This entails avoiding obvious sources of gluten, like bread and pasta, but also being aware of hidden gluten in processed foods, medications, and even some personal care products. Effective management of celiac disease requires learning to read labels, ask questions, and stand up for oneself.

SIGNS AND PROGNOSIS

The symptoms of celiac disease can be mild, moderate, severe, or affect different systems of the body. Symptoms that are commonly associated with the digestive system include nausea, diarrhea, constipation, bloating, and abdominal pain.

These symptoms can be mistaken for other gastrointestinal disorders, like irritable bowel syndrome (IBS). Symptoms that are not related to the digestive system include fatigue, joint pain, headaches, and skin rashes, particularly dermatitis herpetiformis, which is a blistering, itchy skin condition.

To make the diagnosis of celiac disease, a small sample of tissue is taken from the small intestine during a biopsy, which looks for damage to the villi, the tiny finger-like projections that line the intestine and absorb nutrients. Blood tests look for specific antibodies that are usually present in people with celiac disease. If these tests suggest celiac disease, a biopsy is often performed to confirm the diagnosis.

If celiac disease is not treated, the ongoing damage to the small intestine can result in malnutrition, an increased risk of certain cancers, and other autoimmune disorders. For this reason, anyone with a family history of celiac disease or who has persistent symptoms should see a healthcare professional for appropriate testing and diagnosis as soon as possible to prevent long-term health complications associated with celiac disease.

Because gluten causes damage to the small intestine, the body is unable to absorb vital vitamins and minerals, which can result in deficiencies. Iron, calcium, vitamin D, and B vitamins are among the most commonly deficient nutrients in people with celiac disease, and these deficiencies can lead to anemia, osteoporosis, and neurological problems. Celiac disease has a major impact on overall health because of this.

Apart from malnutrient shortages, other illnesses that can be brought on by celiac disease include osteoporosis (from calcium and vitamin D malabsorption), infertility and miscarriages, neurological conditions like peripheral neuropathy and ataxia, and even some cancers, like small bowel lymphoma.

The long-term inflammatory and immunological reaction that gluten causes can also lead to other autoimmune diseases, like type 1 diabetes and thyroid issues.

Maintaining a strict gluten-free diet is crucial for managing celiac disease and preventing these complications. Following the diet helps the small intestine heal, enhances nutrient absorption, lowers the risk of related health conditions, relieves symptoms, and improves the overall quality of life for those who have the disease. Dietitians and healthcare providers can be consulted regularly to monitor health and ensure dietary compliance.

THE VALUE OF DIETARY MANAGEMENT

The foundation of celiac disease treatment is diet management. The main objective is to remove all gluten from the diet to facilitate the healing of the small intestine and avoid future damage. This includes avoiding obvious gluten-containing foods like bread, pasta, and cereals as well as being aware of hidden sources of gluten in processed foods, sauces, and even medications.

A gluten-free diet necessitates substantial lifestyle adjustments as well as continuous awareness. One must carefully read food labels and be mindful of cross-contamination, which happens when gluten-free foods come into contact with gluten-containing foods during processing or preparation. Traveling and eating out can also provide difficulties, so it's important to plan and let restaurant staff know about any dietary requirements you may have.

To maintain a healthy and nutritious gluten-free diet, people with celiac disease can benefit greatly from the information, recipes, and support those dietitians, healthcare professionals, and support groups can offer. By managing their condition appropriately and with the right help, people with celiac disease can live long, pain-free lives.

GLUTEN'S PART IN CELIAC DISEASE

The protein gluten, which is present in wheat, barley, and rye, sets off an immune reaction in people who have celiac disease. When a person with celiac disease eats gluten, their immune system misinterprets the lining of their small intestine, resulting in inflammation and damage to the villi. The villi are important for the absorption of nutrients, and damage to them causes the various symptoms and complications that come with the condition.

To manage celiac disease and prevent damage to the intestines, one must avoid gluten. This includes avoiding bread, pasta, pastries, and cereals made from wheat, barley, or rye.

It also means being aware of gluten in less obvious places, like sauces, soups, salad dressings, and processed foods. There are a variety of gluten-free options available, such as bread, pasta, and baked goods made from grains like rice, corn, and quinoa.

For those with celiac disease, knowing how gluten plays a part in the condition is essential. It enables them to make proactive dietary decisions and avoid gluten exposure. Knowledge and awareness regarding gluten sources and cross-contamination are essential for successful management and maintaining good health.

Armed with the right information and resources, people with celiac disease can successfully manage their dietary restrictions and take advantage of a wide range of safe, gluten-free foods.

CHAPTER TWO

ADVANTAGES OF A DIET FREE OF GLUTEN

The benefits of a gluten-free diet are numerous, especially for those with celiac disease or gluten sensitivity. The diet excludes gluten, a protein present in wheat, barley, and rye that can cause negative reactions in sensitive individuals. The main advantage of a gluten-free diet is the reduction of symptoms like diarrhea, constipation, bloating, and abdominal pain. The healing of the intestines caused by avoiding gluten results in better nutrient absorption and overall digestive health. Moreover, many individuals who follow a gluten-free diet report feeling more energized and having clearer thoughts.

Another important benefit is the reduction of inflammation. People with celiac disease often have inflammation in the small intestine, which can cause long-term damage if not managed. Removing gluten reduces the inflammatory response, which can also lower the risk of other autoimmune conditions that are frequently linked to celiac disease, like thyroid disorders and Type 1 diabetes. The diet can also have a positive effect on the skin, improving conditions like dermatitis herpetiformis, a skin manifestation of celiac disease.

Many people find that a gluten-free diet improves their mood and mental health. Studies show that gluten may have an impact on the brain, causing neurological symptoms such as headaches, depression, and anxiety in some people. When gluten is eliminated from the diet, these symptoms typically go away and people enjoy a higher quality of life. In addition, following a gluten-free diet can encourage a more mindful way of eating by promoting the consumption of whole, unprocessed foods, which is beneficial for general health and wellness.

TYPICAL SOURCES OF GLUTEN

To effectively follow a gluten-free diet, it is important to know what common sources of gluten there are.

Generally speaking, gluten is found in wheat, barley, and rye, as well as any food made from these grains. This includes obvious products like bread, pasta, cereals, and baked goods, but it can also be found in less obvious products like soups, sauces, salad dressings, and even processed meats because these products use wheat-based thickeners or fillers.

Cross-contaminated foods are another common source of gluten. Cross-contamination happens when gluten-free foods come into contact with gluten-containing foods during processing, packaging, or cooking. For example, oats are naturally gluten-free, but they are frequently processed in facilities that handle wheat, which can contaminate them. To make sure packaged foods adhere to strict gluten-free standards, look for certified gluten-free labels.

Gluten can also be found in a variety of food additives and ingredients that go by different names. Some examples of these hidden sources of gluten are malt flavoring, hydrolyzed vegetable protein, and modified food starch. It's important to be aware of these sources and to read food labels carefully. Eating out can also present challenges because gluten can be found in marinades and sauces and as a contaminant on kitchen surfaces and utensils. It's also important to be clear with restaurant staff about dietary restrictions.

RISKS OF CROSS-CONTAMINATION

Cross-contamination is a major concern for people on a gluten-free diet because even minute amounts of gluten can trigger symptoms in those who are sensitive. Cross-contamination happens when gluten-free food comes into contact with gluten-containing food, either directly or indirectly, during food preparation, cooking, or serving. Examples of cross-contamination include using the same toaster for regular and gluten-free bread or not cleaning the kitchen thoroughly after handling gluten-containing food.

Maintaining a designated gluten-free area in the kitchen, using separate cutting boards, utensils, and cookware for gluten-free foods, storing gluten-free foods in distinct containers with clear labeling, keeping a dedicated gluten-free toaster, and avoiding double-dipping (which can introduce gluten particles into the container) are all important ways to reduce the risks of cross-contamination at home.

Choose restaurants that have a dedicated gluten-free menu or are known for their attention to dietary restrictions. Being proactive and informed can significantly reduce the risk of cross-contamination and ensure a safe dining experience. When dining out or ordering food, it's crucial to communicate the need for a strict gluten-free meal to restaurant staff. Ask about the restaurant's practices for preventing cross-contamination, such as using separate fryers or grills for gluten-free foods.

EXAMINING NUTRITION LABELS

Food labels provide information about the ingredients used in the product; it's important to look for any mention of wheat, barley, rye, or related grains. Many countries have regulations requiring allergens, including gluten, to be listed on food labels, which aids in identifying safe products. Reading food labels is an essential skill for anyone following a gluten-free diet.

Some labels will specifically state if the product is gluten-free, but if in doubt, it's best to contact the manufacturer directly to confirm the product's gluten-free status. Look for certifications from reputable organizations that ensure that the product meets strict gluten-free standards.

Ingredients that can contain gluten but may not be immediately recognizable as such, such as malt flavoring, hydrolyzed vegetable protein, and modified food starch, can contain gluten.

Learning to effectively read labels will help ensure that the foods consumed are genuinely gluten-free and safe for people with celiac disease or gluten sensitivity. Additionally, some processed foods and additives may not explicitly mention gluten but are made from gluten-containing grains. Terms like "natural flavorings" or "spices" can sometimes hide gluten unless they are specifically stated as gluten-free. It's also important to check for cross-contamination warnings, such as "may contain traces of wheat" or "processed in a facility that also processes wheat."

DIETARY CONSIDERATIONS

Because many gluten-containing grains are fortified with nutrients like iron, calcium, and B vitamins, maintaining a balanced and nutritious gluten-free diet requires careful planning to ensure that all essential nutrients are consumed. To make up for this, it's important to include a variety of naturally gluten-free grains and starches in the diet, such as quinoa, rice, buckwheat, and potatoes, which can provide essential nutrients and fiber.

Aside from that, people following a gluten-free diet should concentrate on eating whole, unprocessed foods to guarantee that they are getting enough vitamins and minerals. Rich in vital nutrients and naturally gluten-free, fruits, vegetables, lean proteins, and dairy products can help prevent nutrient deficiencies and support general health. If a person's diet isn't enough to meet their needs, a healthcare professional may advise them to consider taking gluten-free vitamin and mineral supplements.

Prioritizing whole foods and being aware of nutrient intake can help people on a gluten-free diet maintain optimal health and well-being while effectively managing their gluten sensitivity or celiac disease. It's also important to keep an eye out for potential over-reliance on gluten-free processed foods, which can be high in sugar, fat, and calories but low in essential nutrients.

CHAPTER THREE

CRUCIAL ELEMENTS OF A CELIAC DIET

FREE OF GLUTEN GRAINS AND FLOUR

A staple of a celiac diet is gluten-free grains and flour, which can be used as a base for a variety of recipes. Quinoa, for example, can be used in salads, as a side dish, or even baked; rice, particularly brown rice, has fiber and can be used in stir-fries, desserts, and many other recipes; and millet, which is sometimes forgotten, can be a hearty breakfast choice or a casserole base.

Among flours, gluten-free substitutes like almond flour, coconut flour, and buckwheat flour are invaluable. Almond flour works wonders in baking, lending a moist texture and nutty flavor to cakes and cookies.

Coconut flour, with its high fiber content, is ideal for recipes calling for a denser texture, like muffins and bread. Buckwheat flour, true to its name, is gluten-free and works wonders for pancakes and crepes.

Try experimenting with these gluten-free grains and flours to maintain culinary creativity while guaranteeing that meals for people with celiac disease remain safe and nutritious. You can mix and match them to create a wide variety of tastes and textures that make following a gluten-free diet less restrictive.

SAFE THICKENERS AND STARCHES

Thickness and starches are essential in gluten-free cooking because they give soups, baked goods, and sauces the proper consistency. Common safe starches are potato starch, tapioca starch, and cornstarch. Cornstarch is great for thickening soups and sauces because it adds a smooth texture without changing the flavor. Tapioca starch is great for thickening and baking because it gives baked goods a chewy texture and sauces a glossy finish.

Another gluten-free option is potato starch, which is great for baking because it gives cakes and breads moisture and a soft texture; it's also great for frying to get a crispy coating.

When using these starches, it's important to remember that a little goes a long way because they are very effective and can thicken liquids quickly when heated.

Apart from these starches, other common thickeners found in gluten-free recipes are xanthan gum and guar gum. These gums are used in small amounts to improve the texture and structure of baked goods, making sure they hold together well and don't crumble.

They help mimic the elasticity and chewiness that gluten provides, making them essential in gluten-free baking.

DAIRY AND ALTERNATIVES TO DAIRY

Dairy products are a good source of calcium and vitamin D, but there are many other options available for people with celiac disease who also have lactose intolerance or who would rather avoid dairy. If dairy products are gluten-free, they can be consumed, but many people choose to use dairy substitutes like almond milk, coconut milk, and soy milk.

Almond milk is a widely used substitute for regular milk because of its mild flavor and versatility in both sweet and savory dishes. It works well for baking, smoothies, and as a milk substitute in coffee or cereal. Coconut milk is rich and creamy and works well for curries, soups, and desserts. Another popular substitute is soy milk, which has a high protein content and can be used in recipes and beverages just like regular milk.

Not only are there milk substitutes but also dairy-free cheese and yogurt options available. Nutritional yeast can be used to replace cheese in salads and pasta dishes to give them a cheesy flavor without containing dairy products.

Almond, coconut, or soy milk can be used to make dairy-free yogurt that can be used for baking, snacking, or recipes that call for yogurt. These options guarantee that people with celiac disease can still enjoy the flavors and benefits of dairy products without sacrificing their health.

Vegetables like spinach, broccoli, and carrots are versatile and can be included in salads, stir-fries, and soups to ensure a nutrient-rich diet; fresh fruits like apples, berries, and oranges provide natural sweetness and can be enjoyed as snacks, in smoothies, or as part of desserts. Legumes are an important part of a celiac diet, offering a wealth of vitamins, minerals, and fiber.

A mainstay of a gluten-free diet, legumes (beans, lentils, and chickpeas) are great sources of protein and fiber and can be used in a wide range of recipes, from salads and side dishes to hearty stews and soups. For example, black beans can be added to salads or made into a dip, while lentils can be used in soups or as a meat substitute in vegetarian dishes.

Incorporating a diverse array of fruits, vegetables, and legumes into meals not only helps ensure a balanced diet that supports overall health and well-being for those with celiac disease, but these plant-based foods also offer a range of flavors and textures and are naturally gluten-free, making them safe and beneficial choices for anyone following a gluten-free lifestyle.

SPICES, HERBS, AND ADDITIVES

Fresh herbs like basil, cilantro, and parsley can lift the flavor of salads, sauces, and main dishes. Basil, for example, is great for making pesto or adding to tomato-based dishes; cilantro can add a fresh, zesty note to salsas and Asian cuisine; parsley is versatile and can be used in almost any dish for a fresh, vibrant flavor. Herbs, spices, and flavorings are essential in adding depth and complexity to gluten-free dishes, eliminating the need for gluten-containing ingredients.

Paprika adds a smoky flavor that's great for seasoning meats and stews; turmeric, with its unique color and health benefits, can be used in curries, rice dishes, and even smoothies for an anti-inflammatory boost; and cumin, which adds warmth and earthiness to dishes like chili and roasted vegetables, is a must-have when cooking gluten-free.

Flavorings such as ginger, lemon zest, and vanilla extract are essential for making delectable gluten-free dishes and desserts. Ground or fresh ginger adds a spicy kick to stir-fries, soups, and baked goods. Experimenting with these herbs, spices, and flavorings can make gluten-free cooking interesting and tasty, guaranteeing that meals are anything but boring.

CHAPTER FOUR

SETTING UP A KITCHEN FOR A GLUTEN-FREE DIET

HOW TO ARRANGE YOUR KITCHEN

Putting your kitchen for a gluten-free diet begins with a thorough clean-out. Take out everything that contains gluten, including bread, pasta, wheat flour, and snacks. If anyone in the house still eats these items, throw them out or put them in a different area. Wipe out all surfaces, utensils, and appliances thoroughly to remove any traces of gluten. Setting aside a specific area in your kitchen for gluten avoidance helps prevent cross-contamination and ensures a safe cooking environment.

Next, separate gluten-free from gluten-containing items in your pantry, refrigerator, and cupboards. Set aside specific shelves or sections for gluten-free products to reduce the possibility of mix-ups. Think about color-coding containers or using labels to distinguish gluten-free items easily. Next, categorize and store gluten-free items in clearly labeled containers.

Use airtight containers to keep gluten-free flours, grains, and snacks fresh and uncontaminated.

Keeping gluten-free utensils, cutting boards, and baking supplies in a separate drawer or cabinet will help you organize your cooking area and make preparing gluten-free meals easier.

GLUTEN-FREE KITCHEN UTENSILS AND APPLIANCES

To keep your gluten-free kitchen safe, it's important to invest in specialized cooking tools and gadgets. Start with the basics: knives, cutting boards, and mixing bowls. To avoid cross-contamination, use separate cutting boards for gluten-free foods. Glass or stainless steel mixing bowls are better than plastic ones because they are easier to clean.

Think about specialized appliances like a gluten-free bread maker and toaster. Ordinary toasters can trap gluten crumbs, which makes it hard to make fully gluten-free toast. A specialized toaster guarantees that your toast stays clean.

A gluten-free bread maker lets you make gluten-free bread without having to worry about cross-contamination from past baked goods.

Invest in tools that make cooking gluten-free easier, like food processors, silicone baking mats, and measuring cups and spoons. When baking gluten-free, exact ingredient measurements are necessary to get the right texture. Silicone baking mats are easy to clean and prevent sticking, and a food processor can help make gluten-free flours and doughs. Make sure to periodically check and clean these tools to make sure they stay gluten-free.

STEER CLEAR OF CROSS-CONTAMINATION

For anyone with celiac disease or gluten sensitivity, preventing cross-contamination is essential. To start, follow stringent kitchen hygiene procedures: wash your hands well before handling gluten-free ingredients; wipe down all surfaces, utensils, and appliances both before and after use; and use different sponges and dishcloths for cleaning gluten-containing and gluten-free items.

Establish stringent segregation procedures when preparing food. Set aside particular cookware, cutting boards, and utensils for use in gluten-free cooking. Wooden utensils and cutting boards should be avoided because they can retain gluten even after washing; instead, use stainless steel, silicone, or glass substitutes that are easier to clean thoroughly. Store gluten-containing and gluten-free products in distinct, labeled spaces to avoid unintentional confusion.

Apart from physical separation, be aware of gluten particles in the air. When using gluten-free flours in baking, handle them carefully to prevent fine particles from being dispersed. Wipe down surfaces with a damp cloth to prevent gluten dust from settling.

KEEPING INGREDIENTS FREE OF GLUTEN

For gluten-free flours, grains, and snacks, use airtight containers to keep them fresh and free from moisture. Label each container clearly with the contents and date of storage to monitor freshness and avoid confusion. Store these containers in a designated gluten-free area of your pantry or kitchen to prevent mix-ups. Proper storage is essential to maintaining the quality and preventing contamination of gluten-free ingredients.

Use vacuum-sealed bags or airtight containers for freezing, and label them with the date to ensure proper rotation and usage. Many gluten-free flours, like almond flour and coconut flour, have higher fat content and spoil quickly at room temperature. To extend their shelf life, store them in the refrigerator or freezer.

Clearly label products to prevent cross-contamination; designate shelves or sections for gluten-free ingredients; clean these areas frequently to maintain a safe storage environment; and teach all family members about these storage practices to ensure everyone follows the same guidelines, maintaining a gluten-free kitchen.

TIPS FOR MEAL PLANNING AND PREPARATION

The secret to sticking to a gluten-free diet is to prepare and plan your meals well. Begin by making a weekly meal plan with a range of gluten-free recipes.

Center your meals around naturally gluten-free foods such as fruits, vegetables, meats, and gluten-free grains. This will help you eat less processed gluten-free food and maintain a balanced diet.

Cooking in bulk and freezing meals can save time and guarantee that you always have gluten-free options available. Label frozen meals with the date and contents for easy identification and rotation. Wash, chop, and store vegetables in airtight containers. Pre-cook grains like quinoa or rice.

Maintain a list of your go-to gluten-free recipes and ingredients to make grocery shopping easier. Utilize gluten-free cookbooks and online resources for meal inspiration and variety. Regularly review and update your meal plans to include new recipes and seasonal ingredients. Keep your pantry stocked with necessary gluten-free staples like gluten-free flour, pasta, and snacks.

CHAPTER FIVE

MAKING THE SWITCH TO A GLUTEN-FREE DIET

HOW TO MAKE A TRANSITION

Starting a gluten-free diet involves going through your pantry and throwing out anything that contains gluten, like bread, pasta, cereals, and snacks made of wheat, barley, and rye. You should also replace these items with gluten-free alternatives like rice, quinoa, gluten-free oats, and gluten-free pasta. You should also make sure that any naturally occurring gluten-free foods you store are free of contamination from processing, such as fruits, vegetables, meat, fish, and dairy products.

Next, create new cooking habits to prevent cross-contamination: use toasters, cutting boards, and cooking utensils specifically for gluten-free foods; thoroughly clean surfaces before starting any meal preparation; and teach family members about the significance of keeping gluten-containing and gluten-free foods apart.

Try out different gluten-free recipes to find tasty meals that suit your new diet. Getting a few gluten-free cookbooks can help inspire you and make the transition easier.

Joining a local or online gluten-free community can offer additional advice and support as you adjust to your new lifestyle. Another important step is learning how to successfully navigate grocery stores. While many stores have designated sections for gluten-free products, it's important to know how to find and choose safe products throughout the store. Gluten-free labels can be helpful but always double-check ingredient lists. Familiarize yourself with gluten-free grains and flours, such as almond flour, coconut flour, and chickpea flour, and incorporate them into your baking and cooking.

HANDLING TEMPTATIONS AND CRAVINGS

One of the most difficult aspects of going gluten-free is managing cravings for gluten-containing foods. To start, try finding satisfying gluten-free alternatives to your favorite foods.

For example, if you miss pizza, try making or purchasing a gluten-free crust. If you have a craving for baked goods, look up recipes for gluten-free bread, cakes, and cookies. Having a variety of gluten-free snacks on hand can also help quell cravings when they arise.

Focusing on the abundance of naturally gluten-free foods is another useful tactic. You should also rediscover the delights of eating fresh fruits, vegetables, nuts, seeds, and lean proteins. You should also try new recipes and cuisines, like Thai or Mexican, that traditionally use gluten-free ingredients. All of these will help you overcome cravings and expand your palate, as well as improve the enjoyment of your diet.

The psychological side of cravings must also be addressed. Remind yourself of the health advantages of a gluten-free diet, particularly if you have celiac disease or gluten sensitivity. Track your cravings and identify triggers by keeping a food journal. Eventually, your body will adjust to the new diet, and cravings will lessen. Ask for help from friends, family, or support groups to help you through this difficult part of the transition.

DINING OUT AND SOCIAL OCCURRENCES

When you follow a gluten-free diet, going to social events and eating out can be challenging, but with a little planning and research, you can enjoy these occasions without jeopardizing your health. Many restaurants now offer gluten-free menus or can accommodate special dietary requests.

If in doubt, call ahead to discuss your needs with the staff and make sure they understand the importance of avoiding cross-contamination.

If you have dietary restrictions, let the host know in advance and offer to bring a gluten-free dish to share so you have something to eat. Potlucks and buffets can be tricky, so it's a good idea to eat a small meal before to avoid being overly full and tempted by unhealthy foods.

Get knowledgeable about ingredients and preparation techniques and don't be afraid to speak up for your health.

Carrying a travel card that explains your dietary requirements in the local language can be quite helpful when dining out in foreign countries. Traveling while gluten-free requires extra planning, but it's completely doable. Bring gluten-free snacks for the journey and research your destination to find gluten-free restaurants and grocery stores. Many countries have gluten-free apps and resources to help you navigate local cuisine safely.

MENTAL AND EMOTIONAL ASSISTANCE

Finding emotional and psychological support is essential to help you manage these changes. To start, educate yourself about celiac disease or gluten sensitivity so that you can better understand your condition and the necessity of your new diet. Knowledge empowers you to make informed decisions and feel more in control.

Making the switch to a gluten-free lifestyle can be emotionally taxing, especially if you feel alone or overwhelmed.

Developing a support network of friends and family who are aware of your dietary needs can also make a big difference. Don't be afraid to communicate your feelings and seek their understanding and assistance. Joining local or online support groups for people with celiac disease or gluten sensitivity offers a platform to share your feelings, exchange tips, and receive encouragement from those who understand your challenges. Connecting with others who share your experience can provide significant emotional support.

Healthy coping strategies are crucial for handling stress and emotions. Regular exercise can improve your mood and general well-being. Mindfulness, meditation, or yoga can help you manage stress and keep a positive outlook. If you find the transition especially difficult, think about getting professional assistance from a therapist who specializes in chronic illness or diet-related issues. They can offer strategies and support to help you navigate the emotional aspects of your new lifestyle.

LOCATING RESOURCES AND SUPPORT GROUPS THAT ARE GLUTEN-FREE

To ensure a successful transition to a gluten-free lifestyle, it is essential to locate trustworthy gluten-free resources and support groups. Begin by investigating reputable websites and organizations that are devoted to celiac disease and gluten sensitivity. These sources frequently offer thorough information on gluten-free diets, recipes, product reviews, and the most recent research. Make sure to bookmark these sites and visit them frequently for advice and inspiration.

Books and cookbooks about living a gluten-free lifestyle are great resources. Look for well-reviewed books with meal plans, helpful advice, and delicious recipes. These books can help you develop a well-stocked gluten-free kitchen and learn about new foods and cooking methods.

You can also stay up to date on new products, trends, and advice from professionals in the field by subscribing to gluten-free magazines or newsletters.

Whether you attend in-person or virtually, support groups can give you a sense of belonging and a common experience. Discussion boards, social media groups, and local gatherings are places where you can ask questions, share your story, and get advice from people who have been through similar experiences. These groups can also share helpful resources like brands that are gluten-free, restaurant recommendations, and social media etiquette advice. By interacting with these communities, you can help your transition go more smoothly and enjoy it more.

CHAPTER SIX

GLUTEN-FREE PASTRIES AND BREADS

Almond flour, coconut flour, or gluten-free all-purpose flour blends are some of the alternative flours that can be used to make gluten-free bread. To make a light and fluffy loaf of gluten-free bread, combine your selected flour with a binder such as xanthan gum to simulate the elasticity that gluten provides. Then, mix in yeast, warm water, and a small amount of sugar to activate the yeast. Let the dough rise in a warm location before baking it in a preheated oven until it is golden brown. For pastries, use the same flour substitutes along with ingredients like dairy-free butter, eggs, and a sweetener. Chilling the dough before baking can help the dough achieve the desired texture.

To make wonderful gluten-free muffins or scones, mix your gluten-free flour with baking powder, a small pinch of salt, and your favorite flavorings, such as chocolate chips or blueberries. Keeping the proper moisture balance is important, so thoroughly combine wet ingredients (milk or almond milk, eggs, and oil) with the dry ingredients before adding them to the dry mixture. Pour the batter into muffin tins or form it into scones, and bake until a toothpick inserted into the center comes out clean.

You can also experiment with different recipes to get delicious results, like gluten-free cinnamon rolls or croissants. These usually call for a little more skill, like rolling and folding to make layers. You should also be patient with the dough, giving it enough time to rise and rest so that it develops the best flavor and texture. With some practice, you'll be able to enjoy a variety of baked goods that are gluten-free and ideal for breakfast or any time of the day.

JUICES AND SMOOTHIES

Smoothies and juices provide a high-nutrient, fast way to start the day—especially for people with celiac disease.

To start, choose fresh, gluten-free fruits and vegetables. To make a traditional green smoothie, combine spinach, kale, or avocado with a banana, some berries, and a liquid base like almond milk or coconut water. You can also add a spoonful of chia or flaxseeds for extra fiber and omega-3 fatty acids. The finished beverage is creamy and satisfying and can be customized with protein powder or nut butter for more protein.

Use complementary fruits and vegetables to create a refreshing juice. For example, a simple yet delicious combination could be apples, carrots, and ginger. Run these through a juicer, or if you don't have one, you can use a high-speed blender with a small amount of water. Then, strain the mixture through cheesecloth or a fine mesh sieve.

The key is to balance the flavors so that you have a good balance of sweetness and tanginess. These kinds of juices are not only delicious but also nutrient-dense.

Aim for fresh, seasonal produce to maximize flavor and nutritional benefits, making each smoothie or juice a powerhouse of gluten-free goodness. Experimenting with different combinations can keep your morning routine exciting.

For example, try blending tropical fruits like mango and pineapple with coconut milk for a taste of the tropics or creating a berry blend with strawberries, raspberries, and blueberries. Adding greens like cucumber or celery to your juice can boost hydration and nutrients.

GRANOLAS AND CEREALS

With a little imagination and the right ingredients, it's easy to make cereals and granolas gluten-free. To make granola, combine gluten-free oats with nuts, seeds, and a sweetener like honey or maple syrup; spread onto a baking sheet and bake at a low temperature, stirring occasionally, until golden and crunchy. You can also add flavor by adding dried fruits, coconut flakes, or spices like nutmeg or cinnamon.

Making your gluten-free cereals is just as easy and satisfying. Toss your favorite nuts and seeds with some gluten-free puffed rice or quinoa. Toast them gently in the oven and top with a little honey and sea salt for a crunchy and tasty breakfast option. Keep your cereal fresh in an airtight container and serve it with your favorite dairy-free milk.

Make a batch of gluten-free oatmeal for a hot breakfast option. Cook the gluten-free oats in water or milk, then stir in fruits (bananas or apples), nut butter, and a dash of cinnamon. This warm, comforting meal comes together quickly and can be customized with different toppings to suit your preferences. You can make your cereals and granolas, which will guarantee that they are healthy and safe for a gluten-free diet.

EGG-BASED RECIPES

Egg-based breakfast recipes are naturally gluten-free and incredibly versatile. Begin your day with a basic scramble, which is made by whisking eggs with a little milk or water and cooking over medium heat, stirring occasionally. To add extra flavor and nutrients, add veggies like spinach, tomatoes, or bell peppers. To up the protein content, add cheese or cooked meats like ham or bacon.

Another flexible option is omelets. Beat the eggs and transfer them to a heated, oiled pan. When the edges begin to set, add your fillings. Fold the omelet in half and cook until the eggs are set through. There are countless options for fillings, from traditional ham and cheese to more daring options like smoked salmon and cream cheese or sautéed mushrooms and feta. Omelets are quick, filling, and simple to tailor to your pantry's contents.

Egg-based dishes are a great choice for a gluten-free diet, offering high-quality protein and endless possibilities to keep breakfast interesting. For a make-ahead option, try egg muffins or a frittata. Whisk a dozen eggs with your favorite mix-ins like vegetables, meats, and cheeses. Pour the mixture into a greased muffin tin or a baking dish, then bake until fully set and golden. These can be refrigerated and reheated throughout the week for a quick and wholesome breakfast.

SIMPLE AND FAST BREAKFAST RECIPES

Quick and simple gluten-free breakfast recipes come in handy on hectic mornings. One such recipe is overnight oats, which you can customize with shredded coconut, chia seeds, or cocoa powder for some variation. Simply combine gluten-free oats with milk or a dairy-free substitute, add a sweetener like honey or maple syrup, and top with fruits and nuts. Set it in the refrigerator overnight to have a wholesome breakfast that's ready to eat in the morning.

Another quick and healthy option is smoothie bowls, which are made by blending a thick smoothie base with frozen fruits, a few greens, and a splash of liquid. Then, pour the mixture into a bowl and top with granola, fresh fruit, and a drizzle of nut butter. The thick consistency combined with the assortment of toppings makes this a filling meal that feels more substantial than a typical smoothie, and it's simple to customize to your tastes.

If you'd prefer a savory breakfast, toast a slice of gluten-free bread and top it with avocado and a poached egg. Sprinkle with salt, pepper, and a squeeze of lemon juice for a quick, satisfying meal. These quick and easy recipes ensure you can enjoy a delicious gluten-free breakfast even on the busiest mornings. You can also make a yogurt parfait, which is even simpler: layer gluten-free yogurt with fresh fruits, gluten-free granola, and a drizzle of honey. This can be put together in a matter of minutes and offers a balanced mix of protein, carbohydrates, and healthy fats.

WRAPS AND SANDWICHES

Choosing the right ingredients and putting them together in a creative way is the key to making delicious and gluten-free sandwiches and wraps. To start, start with gluten-free bread or wraps made from ingredients like rice flour, quinoa flour, or almond flour, which are easily found in many grocery stores. For fillings, go for protein-rich options like grilled chicken, turkey, or tofu, paired with fresh vegetables and spreads like avocado or hummus. An important tip for creating delicious gluten-free sandwiches and wraps is to use layers of different veggies, like lettuce, tomatoes, and cucumbers, to add flavor and crunch. Finally, roll or fold the wrap tightly to make sure it stays together well.

Try varying the flavors and textures in your lunches to keep things interesting. For example, a Mediterranean-style wrap could have grilled chicken, feta cheese, spinach, and sun-dried tomatoes with balsamic vinegar and olive oil drizzle.

Another option is to make a traditional turkey and avocado sandwich on gluten-free bread and top it with mashed avocado, sliced turkey breast, lettuce, and a dash of salt and pepper. These options are not only great for people who have celiac disease but also offer a filling and healthy lunch option for anyone looking to eat gluten-free.

DRESSINGS AND SALADS

Salads are a great way to add variety and boost protein content. Start with a base of fresh greens like spinach, kale, or mixed lettuce. Add a variety of colorful vegetables like bell peppers, carrots, and cherry tomatoes for crunch and nutrition. You can also add sources of protein like grilled chicken, chickpeas, or quinoa.

Make your dressings to keep your salad gluten-free. Easy vinaigrette to make is just olive oil, vinegar (like balsamic or apple cider), Dijon mustard, and a little honey or maple syrup for sweetness. Shake or whisk together until emulsified, then drizzle over your salad.

If you're in the mood for something heftier, try making gluten-free pasta salads with brown rice or quinoa pasta. Once cooked, toss with diced vegetables, herbs, and a homemade dressing for a light and satisfying meal. Grain-free salads, such as this one made with quinoa, roasted vegetables, and lemon tahini dressing; make a filling and healthy lunch option that can be adjusted to accommodate different dietary needs and allergies.

STEWS AND SOUPS

Comforting, hot soups and stews are great options for gluten-free lunches, especially in the winter. Start with a gluten-free stock or broth as the foundation; common choices are vegetable broth, chicken broth, or bone broth. Add substantial veggies like potatoes, carrots, and celery, as well as proteins like beans, lentils, or chicken. Add herbs and spices like thyme, rosemary, and garlic to enhance flavors. Simmer everything until the vegetables are soft and the flavors combine.

Use substitutes like pureed veggies, cornstarch, or arrowroot powder to thicken gluten-free soups.

For instance, pureed squash and coconut milk can thicken a creamy butternut squash soup. Beef, root vegetables, and a tomato-based sauce can make a hearty stew. To make a satisfying gluten-free lunch, serve soups and stews with gluten-free bread or crackers on the side.

RECIPES FOR GLUTEN-FREE PASTA

Pasta without gluten creates a plethora of options for lunch dishes. Brown rice, quinoa, and chickpeas are just a few of the gluten-free pasta options available. These pasta cook similarly to regular pasta, so follow the cooking instructions on the package, being careful not to overcook to preserve texture. Once cooked, serve the pasta with flavorful sauces like Alfredo, marinara, or pesto, which can all be made gluten-free with a few simple ingredient swaps and adjustments.

Try experimenting with different additions and toppings for your pasta dishes. For example, you can make a gluten-free spaghetti carbonara with gluten-free spaghetti, crispy bacon, eggs, and Parmesan cheese.

Another option is to make a vegetable stir-fry with gluten-free noodles and a vinaigrette dressing. Both of these dishes are satisfying and suitable for people who have dietary sensitivity to gluten.

IDEAS FOR A LIGHT AND HEALTHFUL LUNCH

Alternatively, a cool sushi bowl with sushi rice, seaweed salad, cucumber slices, and sashimi-grade fish offers a gluten-free take on traditional sushi. For those looking for lighter options, there are many delicious and nutritious gluten-free lunch ideas.

Try putting together a colorful Buddha bowl with a variety of gluten-free grains like quinoa, mixed with roasted vegetables, and avocado slices, and a protein source like grilled tofu or salmon. Drizzle with a tahini or yogurt-based dressing for extra taste and creaminess.

Make gluten-free wraps with sliced veggies, leafy greens, and a spread like guacamole or hummus; roll tightly and cut into pinwheels for a portable, nutrient-dense lunch.

Another great option is a smoothie bowl, which combines fruits, vegetables, and protein sources like protein powder or yogurt; topped with gluten-free granola and fresh berries for flavor and texture. These healthy, light lunch options are great for keeping you full all day long without sacrificing flavor or dietary restrictions.

MAIN COURSE RECIPES

Finding delicious gluten-free main course recipes can be a delightful and fulfilling experience. There are many options to choose from, including flavorful vegetarian dishes and hearty meat dishes. Some classics to try include homemade meatballs and gluten-free spaghetti made with gluten-free pasta and a mixture of perfectly seasoned ground meats. Another favorite is pan-seared chicken breasts served with a zesty gluten-free lemon sauce and a side of roasted vegetables for a hearty and satisfying meal. These recipes are not only suitable for people with celiac disease but also appeal to anyone looking for tasty and nutritious dinner options.

SIDE DISHES AND ACCOMPANIMENTS

These are essential components of a well-rounded meal. If you're looking for a gluten-free option, try quinoa pilaf with toasted almonds and mixed herbs, which is a nutrient-dense substitute for traditional grains.

Roasted garlic mashed potatoes, made with dairy-free butter and almond milk, go well with any main course. A crisp spinach and strawberry salad dressed with balsamic vinaigrette adds a vibrant pop of color to the table. These gluten-free side dishes not only improve the dining experience but also accommodate a wide range of preferences and dietary requirements, so they're ideal for get-togethers or family dinners.

ONE-POT MEALS

One-pot meals come in handy for hectic days and can be readily modified to be gluten-free. For example, a tasty gluten-free stir-fry of chicken and vegetables with tamari sauce and sesame oil is a dish that is packed with protein and vegetables. Alternatively, a substantial gluten-free chili made with lean ground turkey, kidney beans, and a blend of spices provides warmth and comfort with each bite. These meals are easy to prepare and require minimal cleanup, so they're perfect for people who want simplicity without sacrificing flavor or nutrition.

These casseroles are easy to customize to suit a variety of dietary preferences and are a hit at family dinners or potlucks. One idea for gluten-free casseroles is a Mexican-inspired dish called Gluten-Free Enchilada Casserole, which consists of layers of corn tortillas, shredded chicken or beans, enchilada sauce, and a sprinkle of dairy-free cheese for a flavorful twist. Another option is a comforting gluten-free lasagna, consisting of homemade marinara sauce, fresh vegetables, and creamy ricotta cheese, all nestled between gluten-free lasagna noodles.

FAMILY-FRIENDLY DINNER IDEAS

It's important to provide options that suit the tastes and dietary requirements of all members of the family. For instance, sweet potato fries tossed in olive oil and sea salt add a nutritious touch to this healthier take on a classic favorite. Another family-friendly option is a gluten-free Hawaiian pizza, which is topped with fresh pineapple, Canadian bacon, and dairy-free cheese on a gluten-free crust. These ideas not only accommodate gluten-free diets but also make sure that family dinners are delicious, well-balanced, and enjoyable for everyone gathered around the table.

These ideas and recipes prioritize taste and nutrition while also trying to make cooking easier, so it's possible to follow a gluten-free diet without sacrificing flavor or variety in meals. All of these ideas and recipes are meant to provide helpful, tasty, and approachable options for people with celiac disease or other dietary restrictions.

FAST SNACK RECIPES

Having gluten-free snack recipes on hand is crucial for controlling hunger in between meals when one is following a gluten-free diet. Nutrient-dense homemade trail mix, which combines gluten-free nuts, seeds, and dried fruits, is a great option. Rice cakes with almond butter and sliced banana are another idea that offers a balance of protein and carbohydrates. If you're craving something savory, gluten-free pretzels dipped in hummus or guacamole can be a satisfying choice. These snacks are easy to put together and provide the necessary nutrients to maintain a steady energy level throughout the day.

GLUTEN-FREE FINGER CUISINE

Gluten-free finger foods are ideal for casual get-togethers or party appetizers. A tasty alternative is the gluten-free mini quiches, which are made with a crust made of almond flour or gluten-free oats and filled with veggies, cheese, and herbs for a flavorful bite-sized treat. Another popular option is the gluten-free chicken tenders, which are coated in a mixture of gluten-free breadcrumbs and herbs and baked until golden and crispy. Vegetable sticks, like carrots, cucumbers, and bell peppers, are a healthy and refreshing finger food that is made without requiring gluten.

OPTIONS FOR HEALTHFUL SNACKS

To manage celiac disease, it's important to choose healthy, gluten-free snacks. Apple slices with nut butter are a simple but satisfying snack that provides a combination of fiber, healthy fats, and protein. Greek yogurt with fresh berries on top is another healthy option that provides probiotics, vitamins, and minerals. Homemade kale chips seasoned with olive oil and sea salt are a savory snack that has a crunchy texture and is high in antioxidants. These snacks not only support overall health but also aid in controlling cravings and sustaining energy levels throughout the day.

A cookbook dedicated to the celiac disease diet would be incomplete without gluten-free dips and spreads. Traditional guacamole, made with ripe avocados, tomatoes, onions, and lime juice, is a flavorful and nutritious dip for gluten-free tortilla chips or vegetable sticks. Tzatziki, a Greek yogurt-based dip flavored with cucumber, garlic, and dill, is another delectable option; it goes well with gluten-free pita bread or as a spread for grilled meats. For a little heat, a homemade salsa made with fresh tomatoes, cilantro, jalapeño peppers, and lime juice gives a vibrant pop to any snack or appetizer spread.

PARTY SNACKS

A variety of appetizers that satisfy different dietary requirements are essential when throwing or attending a gluten-free party. To start, try this visually striking but straightforward gluten-free bruschetta, which is made with toasted gluten-free bread topped with diced tomatoes, garlic, basil, and balsamic vinegar. Another sophisticated option is this cream cheese-stuffed mushroom, which is baked until golden and bubbling and contains cream cheese, herbs, and gluten-free breadcrumbs. Finally, for a cool treat, try this crowd-pleasing shrimp cocktail, which is served with a gluten-free cocktail sauce consisting of ketchup, horseradish, and lemon juice.

GLUTEN-FREE GRAINS AND ALTERNATIVES

Choosing the right flour and substitutes is essential for producing delicious results when baking gluten-free due to celiac disease or gluten sensitivity. While traditional wheat flour contains gluten, which is a protein that gives dough its elasticity and helps baked goods rise, gluten-free alternatives can mimic these qualities with the right combinations.

Common gluten-free flours include rice flour, almond flour, coconut flour, and chickpea flour, each of which has a unique texture and flavor. By blending these flours, you can balance out their individual qualities, improving the texture and flavor of your baked goods. For instance, combining rice flour for structure, almond flour for moisture, and a small amount of tapioca starch for elasticity can replicate the qualities of wheat flour in baked goods.

ADVICE FOR BAKING GLUTEN-FREE SUCCESSFULLY

To ensure that your gluten-free creations turn out perfectly, you must pay close attention to the following details: first, always use certified gluten-free ingredients to prevent cross-contamination; second, add xanthan gum or guar gum to your recipes to mimic the elasticity that gluten provides, enhancing texture and structure; third, increase the leavening agents slightly, such as baking powder or baking soda, to help your baked goods rise properly; and finally, make sure your oven temperature is accurate and pay attention to baking times, as gluten-free batters frequently require shorter baking times or lower temperatures to prevent drying out. Finally, let your baked goods cool.

ROLLS AND BREAD

Since gluten is the protein that gives bread its elasticity and structure, baking gluten-free bread and rolls can be difficult to master. You can make gluten-free bread by combining gluten-free flours, such as sorghum flour, brown rice flour, and tapioca starch; you can also add eggs or a binding agent, such as xanthan gum, to improve texture and moisture retention; for rolls, dividing the dough into smaller portions can help achieve better rise and consistency; using a warm, moist environment during proofing can also increase the yeast activity in gluten-free dough, making for softer, more flavorful bread and rolls. Finally, experimenting with different recipes and methods will help you discover the one that best suits your tastes and dietary requirements.

BROWNIES, COOKIES, AND CAKES

Achieving the desired taste and texture in gluten-free cakes, cookies, and brownies requires careful consideration of ingredients and methods; for cakes, using gluten-free flour blends such as a combination of almond flour and potato starch can provide a moist and tender crumb; for cookies, chilling the dough before baking can help prevent spreading and preserve shape; for brownies, using ingredients like almond flour or oat flour can add richness and texture without compromising flavor; and for brownies, adding natural binders such as mashed bananas or flaxseed meal can improve the structure of gluten-free desserts, guaranteeing they hold together well during baking.

PASTRIES AND PIES

With the right methods and ingredients, gluten-free pies and pastries can be a delightful addition to your baking repertoire. For pie crusts, try using a combination of gluten-free flour like oat flour, tapioca starch, and almond flour for a flaky and flavorful crust. To prevent sticking, chill the dough before rolling it out. For fillings, use fresh fruits and natural thickeners like cornstarch or tapioca flour for a luscious texture without using gluten. For pastries like tarts or turnovers, try varying gluten-free flour combinations to yield crispy, golden shells. Finally, brushing the pastry with an egg wash before baking can enhance its color and shine, making your gluten-free pastries as delicious as they are gluten-free.

CHAPTER SEVEN

LONG-TERM NUTRITIONAL PLANS

Due to celiac disease, maintaining a gluten-free lifestyle necessitates long-term dietary strategies that prioritize avoiding gluten-containing foods while maintaining balanced nutrition. To begin, learn what foods are safe to eat and what should be avoided.

Naturally, gluten-free foods can be the basis of your diet. Include gluten-free grains like rice, quinoa, corn, and gluten-free oats, making sure they are certified gluten-free to prevent cross-contamination.

Meal prep is a great way to keep control over ingredients and lower the chance of contamination during cooking. You can also use gluten-free baking and cooking substitutes like almond flour, coconut flour, and gluten-free baking mixes. Label reading is also important because it teaches you where to find hidden sources of gluten in processed foods, sauces, and condiments.

Take your time discovering new and creative gluten-free recipes so that your meals are always exciting and different. Try foods from other cultures that are recognized for being naturally gluten-free, such as Middle Eastern (quinoa salads), Asian (rice noodles), or Mexican (corn tortillas). Pay attention to foods that are high in nutrients to promote general health and make sure you are getting enough fiber, vitamins, and minerals from your diet.

HANDLING NUTRITIONAL DIFFICULTIES

Changing to a gluten-free diet comes with several obstacles, but these can be overcome with proactive approaches. First and foremost, educate yourself—be aware of the signs of gluten exposure and the significance of adhering strictly to a gluten-free diet. Create a network of family, friends, and medical professionals who can offer support and advice.

To promote understanding and cooperation, it may be necessary to be assertive when communicating dietary needs in social situations. Research restaurants in advance or give the chef a call to inquire about gluten-free options. Be on the lookout for cross-contamination hazards in shared kitchen areas and buffets.

Plan your meals creatively to avoid boredom. Try new recipes and cooking methods to make meals interesting and pleasurable. Stock up on gluten-free snacks to avoid feeling hungry in between meals. Make grocery shopping a ritual that involves reading labels and choosing gluten-free products that have been certified.

KEEPING UP WITH GLUTEN-FREE DEVELOPMENTS

Keeping up with developments in gluten-free products, research, and community support is essential to staying informed about gluten-free trends. Reputable sources like health websites, blogs dedicated to the gluten-free lifestyle, and medical journals should be regularly consulted to stay up to date on new findings and recommendations.

Attending in-person or online support groups can provide valuable firsthand experiences and insights from others who are managing celiac disease.

Keep an eye on certifications and labeling laws to make sure that products meet gluten-free requirements. Keep an eye out for newly released gluten-free products and brands that may provide easy ways to stick to a gluten-free diet. Try new recipes and cooking techniques to expand your cooking skills and accommodate changing dietary requirements.

Talk with celiac disease specialists about new treatments or dietary recommendations that could affect your management strategy. Inform your support group about the latest trends and advancements in the gluten-free lifestyle to promote knowledge and comprehension. Being well-informed gives you the power to make wise decisions and successfully adjust to changes in the gluten-free environment.

Having access to resources and ongoing support is crucial for effectively adhering to a gluten-free lifestyle. Create a support system comprising dietitians, medical professionals, and other celiac disease sufferers. Look for credible online communities, forums, or social media groups where members exchange recipes, advice, and emotional support regarding living a gluten-free lifestyle.

Look into educational resources like podcasts, webinars, and books that offer in-depth information on managing celiac disease and gluten-free nutrition; participate in live or online workshops on label reading, gluten-free cooking, and overcoming social obstacles related to dietary restrictions; use smartphone apps that help you find gluten-free restaurants, identify gluten-free products, and keep track of your shopping list.

Engage in clinical trials or research studies looking into new treatments or dietary strategies for celiac disease.

Be proactive in gaining access to resources and support networks that will help you maintain a healthy and fulfilling gluten-free lifestyle. Stay in regular communication with your healthcare team to monitor nutritional status and address any concerns related to adherence to the gluten-free diet.

COMMON ISSUE TROUBLESHOOTING

Common concerns about a gluten-free diet are addressed with helpful tips and troubleshooting techniques. You will learn the fundamentals of gluten cross-contamination and how to avoid it at home and when dining out. You will also become familiar with the labels and symbols of the gluten-free certification to make sure packaged foods are safe.

Discover how to identify the signs of gluten exposure and create a plan for handling inadvertent consumption that includes monitoring symptoms and staying hydrated. Try different grains and flour blends to see which ones work best in your favorite recipes.

Inform caregivers and family members about the significance of keeping a gluten-free environment and meeting your dietary needs.

Plan for your trip by looking up gluten-free restaurants at your destination and bringing along healthy snacks. Be sure to make your dietary requirements known when you go to social events or get-togethers so that accommodations are made. When faced with new circumstances or difficulties in leading a gluten-free lifestyle, don't be afraid to speak up for yourself.

CHAPTER EIGHT

COMMON CELIAC DISEASE SYMPTOMS

Beyond digestive discomfort, people with celiac disease may also experience fatigue, unexplained weight loss, and nutrient deficiencies due to malabsorption. Skin conditions like dermatitis herpetiformis, joint pain, and even neurological symptoms like headaches or tingling sensations in extremities can also arise. Celiac disease is characterized by a variety of symptoms, ranging from digestive issues to systemic effects. Digestive symptoms frequently include chronic diarrhea, abdominal pain, bloating, and constipation.

If you believe you or someone you know may have celiac disease based on these symptoms, you must visit a healthcare practitioner for a proper diagnosis and help in implementing a gluten-free diet. Knowledge of these symptoms is critical for early detection and management of celiac disease.

The cornerstone of managing celiac disease is adhering to a strict gluten-free diet. The first step in ensuring food is gluten-free is carefully reading labels. Look for products that are specifically labeled as gluten-free, as they are tested to meet regulatory standards for gluten content. Items that are not clearly labeled as gluten-free or that are processed in facilities that also handle gluten-containing foods should be avoided, as cross-contamination can occur.

To avoid unintentional gluten exposure, make sure restaurant or retail staff members are aware of your dietary requirements when you are dining out or shopping.

You can also simplify meal preparation at home by using naturally gluten-free ingredients like fruits, vegetables, lean meats, and gluten-free grains like rice or quinoa.

Even with precautions, accidental gluten consumption can occur. If you think you may have consumed gluten, watch for symptoms like bloating, fatigue, or discomfort in your digestive tract. Drink lots of water to help flush out toxins and ease symptoms. Keep gluten-free snacks or meal replacements on hand for situations when there aren't many safe food options.

Your healthcare provider can guide managing symptoms and may suggest short-term dietary changes or medications to relieve discomfort if symptoms worsen or persist. As always, awareness can be strengthened, and a commitment to a gluten-free lifestyle is reinforced by learning from unintentional exposure.

GLUTEN-FREE ACCREDITATIONS

When choosing packaged foods, ingredients, or supplements, look for reputable gluten-free certifications on product labels, such as the Certified Gluten-Free Seal from groups like the Gluten Intolerance Group (GIG) or the Gluten-Free Certification Organization (GFCO). These certifications certify that products meet strict gluten-free standards and go through ongoing testing to ensure compliance.

Maintain confidence in your dietary choices and support your health goals by buying with confidence knowing that the promises made about gluten-free products are real. You may do this by checking certification databases or reliable sources. You can also stay updated on changes to gluten-free regulations and certifications.

HELPING A RELATIVE AFFECTED BY CELIAC DISEASE

Encouraging open communication about their experiences and challenges with celiac disease, offering empathy and helpful advice. Understanding their dietary needs and creating a safe environment are important aspects of supporting a family member with celiac disease. You should also educate yourself about the gluten-free lifestyle, including reading labels, cooking gluten-free meals, and recognizing symptoms of accidental gluten exposure.

To prevent cross-contamination, separate gluten-free and gluten-containing foods in your kitchen. Choose restaurants that can accommodate special dietary requests or offer gluten-free options when dining together. Celebrate small victories along the way to keep yourself motivated and positive.

Attend support groups or look for online communities for additional guidance and encouragement. By speaking up for their health and well-being, you contribute to a supportive environment that improves their quality of life with celiac disease. Keep up to date on research and treatment options related to celiac disease to provide informed support.

www.ingramcontent.com/pod-product-compliance
Lightning Source LLC
Chambersburg PA
CBHW061253250726
48653CB00002B/639